SIBO DEIT COOKBOOK

30 Easily Digestible Low FODMAP Recipes to Reduce Bacteria Growth and Manage Symptoms (FISH, EGG and MEAT RECIPES)

Lucy Rhodes

TABLE OF CONTENT

INTRODUCTION

SIBO stands for Small Intestinal Bacterial Overgrowth, which is a condition where there is an abnormal increase in the overall bacterial population in the small intestine. This disorder is sometimes referred to as blind loop syndrome. SIBO commonly results when a circumstance, such as surgery or disease, slows the flow of contents in the small intestine, creating a breeding ground for bacteria. Excess bacteria frequently induce diarrhea and may result in weight loss and malnutrition.

SIBO symptoms include loss of appetite, gastrointestinal pain, nausea, bloating, an unpleasant feeling of fullness after eating, diarrhea, accidental weight loss, and malnutrition. People with SIBO may require intramuscular vitamin B-12 injections, as well as oral vitamins, calcium, and iron supplements. A lactose-free diet may also be necessary. Correcting nutritional inadequacies is an important element of SIBO treatment, especially for patients who have lost a lot of weight. Malnutrition can be treated, but the resulting damage is not always reversible. Antibiotics are the initial way to treat bacterial overgrowth, but nutritional support is also important.

For many individuals, dietary modifications become a pivotal aspect of SIBO management, with lactose-free diets often proving instrumental in alleviating symptoms and reducing bacterial proliferation. The journey towards restoring gut health demands a holistic approach, one that encompasses not only the eradication of excess bacteria but also the restoration of nutritional balance and the preservation of gastrointestinal integrity.

This SIBO diet cookbook serves as an invaluable tool in your journey towards managing and maintaining optimal gut health. With its carefully curated selection of recipes and dietary guidelines, this cookbook offers a roadmap to navigating the complexities of Small Intestinal Bacterial Overgrowth (SIBO) with confidence and ease. By adhering to the principles of this SIBO-friendly diet, you can effectively manage symptoms, reduce bacterial overgrowth, and promote healing within the gut.

Central to the effectiveness of this SIBO diet cookbook is its emphasis on low FODMAP (Fermentable Oligosaccharides, Disaccharides, Monosaccharides, and Polyols) foods, which are known to exacerbate symptoms of SIBO. By limiting the intake of these fermentable carbohydrates, you can alleviate bloating, gas, and abdominal discomfort, while simultaneously starving the overgrown bacteria responsible for these symptoms.

Moreover, this SIBO diet cookbook provides practical guidance on meal planning, ingredient substitutions, and culinary techniques tailored to the unique needs of individuals with SIBO. From deliciously simple meals to creative culinary creations, each recipe is crafted to nourish your body, support digestive health, and delight the palate.

Ultimately, this SIBO diet cookbook empowers you to take control of your gut health, offering a wealth of resources and recipes to support you on your journey towards digestive wellness. With its invaluable insights and mouthwatering recipes, this cookbook serves as a trusted companion in the quest for a happy, healthy gut.

'' Transform your plate, transform your health— discover the power of SIBO-friendly cuisine.''

Fish Recipes

Grilled Salmon with Lemon and Dill

Marinate salmon fillets in a mixture of olive oil, lemon juice, and fresh dill, and then grill until flaky and tender.

- Serves: 4
- Prep time: 10 minutes
- Cook time: 10 minutes

Ingredients

- 4 salmon fillets (4-6 oz each)
- 2 tbsp. olive oil
- 2 tbsp. fresh lemon juice
- 1 tbsp. fresh dill, chopped
- Salt and pepper to taste

Nutrition information per serving

- Calories: 280
- Protein: 34g
- Fat: 14g
- Carbohydrates: 0g

Instructions
1. Preheat the grill to medium-high heat.

2. In a small bowl, whisk together olive oil, lemon juice, and dill.

3. Season the salmon fillets with salt and pepper, then brush with the olive oil mixture.

4. Place the salmon on the grill, skin-side down, and cook for 4-5 minutes per side, or until the fish is cooked through and flakes easily with a fork.

5. Serve hot with additional lemon wedges, if desired.

Health benefits: Salmon is an excellent source of omega-3 fatty acids, which have been shown to reduce inflammation and improve heart health.

"Nourish your gut, thrive with this cookbook."

Note___________________________________

____

____

____

____

____

Your

Observation___________________________

____

____

____

____

____

____

Progress

Report_________________________________

____

____

____

____

____

____

Baked Cod with Herbs

Season cod fillets with a blend of fresh herbs such as parsley, chives, and thyme, then bake until the fish is cooked through and flaky.

- Serves: 4
- Prep time: 10 minutes
- Cook time: 15 minutes

Ingredients

- 4 cod fillets (4-6 oz each)
- 2 tbsp. olive oil
- 1 tbsp. fresh parsley, chopped
- 1 tbsp. fresh chives, chopped
- 1 tbsp. fresh thyme, chopped
- Salt and pepper to taste

Nutrition information per serving

- Calories: 170
- Protein: 28g
- Fat: 6g
- Carbohydrates: 0g

Instructions

1. Preheat the oven to 400°F.

2. In a small bowl, mix together olive oil, parsley, chives, and thyme.

3. Season cod fillets with salt and pepper, then brush with the herb mixture.

4. Place the cod in a baking dish and bake for 12-15 minutes, or until the fish is cooked through and flakes easily with a fork.

5. Serve hot with lemon wedges, if desired.

Health benefits: Cod is a lean source of protein and a good source of vitamin B12, which is important for nerve and blood cell health.

"Relief in every recipe, satisfaction in every bite."

Note

Your

Observation

Progress

Report

Pan-Seared Tilapia with Cilantro Lime Butter

Sear tilapia fillets in a skillet and top with zesty cilantro and lime butter for a burst of flavor.

- Serves: 4
- Prep time: 10 minutes
- Cook time: 10 minutes

Ingredients

- 4 tilapia fillets (4-6 oz each)
- 2 tbsp. unsalted butter, softened
- 1 tbsp. fresh cilantro, chopped
- 1 lime, zested and juiced
- Salt and pepper to taste

Nutrition information per serving

- Calories: 200
- Protein: 28g
- Fat: 9g
- Carbohydrates: 1g

Instructions
1. In a small bowl, mix together softened butter, cilantro, lime zest, and lime juice.

2. Season tilapia fillets with salt and pepper.

3. Over medium-high heat, heat a large skillet and add a small amount of oil.

4. Add tilapia fillets to the skillet and cook for 3-4 minutes per side, or until the fish is cooked through and flakes easily with a fork.

5. Serve hot with a dollop of cilantro lime butter on top.

Health benefits: Tilapia is a low-fat source of protein and a good source of selenium, which is important for thyroid function.

"Cooking made easy, relief made tasty."

Note____

____

____

____

____

____

Your

Observation_______________________________________

____

____

____

____

____

____

Progress

Report____

____

____

____

____

____

____

Lemon Garlic Shrimp Skewers

Thread shrimp onto skewers, then brush with a mixture of garlic-infused oil and lemon juice before grilling for a delicious and easy-to-make dish.

- Serves: 4
- Prep time: 10 minutes
- Cook time: 10 minutes

Ingredients

- 1 lb. large shrimp, peeled and deveined
- 2 tbsp. garlic-infused oil
- 2 tbsp. fresh lemon juice
- Salt and pepper to taste

Nutrition information per serving

- Calories: 120
- Protein: 23g
- Fat: 2g
- Carbohydrates: 1g

Instructions

1. Preheat the grill to medium-high heat.

2. Thread shrimp on skewers, leaving a small amount of space between each shrimp.

3. In a small bowl, whisk together the garlic-infused oil and lemon juice.

4. Brush shrimp skewers with the oil mixture and season with salt and pepper.

5. Grill shrimp skewers for 2-3 minutes per side, or until the shrimp are pink and cooked through.

6. Serve hot with additional lemon wedges, if desired.

Health benefits: Shrimp is a low-calorie source of protein and a good source of selenium, which is important for thyroid function.

Eating Healthy is Life

Note

Your

Observation

Progress

Report

Tuna Salad Lettuce Wraps

Mix canned tuna with mayonnaise, diced red bell pepper, and green onions (green parts only) and serve in lettuce cups for a refreshing low FODMAP meal.

- Serves: 4
- Prep time: 10 minutes
- Cook time: 0 minutes

Ingredients

- 2 cans tuna, drained
- 1/4 cup mayonnaise
- 1/4 cup diced red bell pepper
- 2 green onions (green parts only), thinly sliced
- Salt and pepper to taste
- 8 large lettuce leaves

Nutrition information per serving

- Calories: 170
- Protein: 20g
- Fat: 9g
- Carbohydrates: 3g

Instructions

1. In a medium bowl, mix together tuna, mayonnaise, red bell pepper, and green onions.

2. To taste, season with salt and pepper.

3. Spoon tuna salad onto lettuce leaves and wrap tightly.

4. Serve cold.

Health benefits: Tuna is a low-fat source of protein and a good source of vitamin D, which is important for bone health.

"Cook with confidence, eat with joy—find relief and satisfaction in every dish."

Note____

____

____

____

____

____

Your

Observation_______________________________________

____

____

____

____

____

____

Progress

Report_______________________________________

____

____

____

____

____

____

Grilled Swordfish Steaks with Herb Marinade

Marinate swordfish steaks in a blend of olive oil, fresh herbs, and lemon zest, then grill to perfection.

- Serves: 4
- Prep time: 10 minutes
- Cook time: 10 minutes

Ingredients

- 4 swordfish steaks (4-6 oz each)
- 2 tbsp. olive oil
- 1 tbsp. fresh parsley, chopped
- 1 tbsp fresh thyme, chopped
- 1 tbsp. fresh rosemary, chopped
- Salt and pepper to taste

Nutrition information per serving

- Calories: 240
- Protein: 34g
- Fat: 11g
- Carbohydrates: 0g

Instructions

1. Preheat the grill to medium-high heat.

2. In a small bowl, mix together olive oil, parsley, thyme, and rosemary.

3. Season swordfish steaks with salt and pepper, then brush with the herb mixture.

4. Place swordfish on the grill and cook for 4-5 minutes per side, or until the fish is cooked through and flakes easily with a fork.

5. Serve hot with lemon wedges, if desired.

Health benefits: Swordfish is a good source of omega-3 fatty acids, which have been shown to reduce inflammation and improve heart health.

Note

Your

Observation

Progress

Report

Baked Haddock with Tomato and Olive Salsa

Top haddock filets with a homemade salsa made from diced tomatoes, olives, and fresh herbs, then bake until the fish is flaky and the salsa is bubbly.

- Serves: 4
- Prep time: 10 minutes
- Cook time: 15 minutes

Ingredients

- 4 haddock fillets (4-6 oz each)
- 2 tbsp. olive oil
- 1 pint cherry tomatoes
- 1/4 cup pitted kalamata olives, chopped
- 1 tbsp. fresh parsley, chopped
- Salt and pepper to taste.

Nutrition information per serving

- Calories: 170
- Protein: 28g
- Fat: 6g
- Carbohydrates: 4g

Instructions

1. Preheat the oven to 400°F.

2. In a small bowl, mix together olive oil, cherry tomatoes, kalamata olives, and parsley.

3. Season haddock fillets with salt and pepper, then place in a baking dish.

4. Spoon the tomato and olive mixture over the haddock fillets.

5. Bake for 12-15 minutes or until the fish is thoroughly cooked and readily flaked with a fork.

6. Serve hot.

Health benefits: Haddock is a lean source of protein and a good source of vitamin B12, which is important for nerve and blood cell health.

Note_______________________________________

____

____

____

____

____

Your

Observation_________________________________

____

____

____

____

____

____

Progress

Report_____________________________________

____

____

____

____

____

Seared Mahi-Mahi with Pineapple Salsa

Sear mahi-mahi fillets in a hot skillet and serve with a vibrant pineapple salsa for a tropical twist.

- Serves: 4
- Prep time: 10 minutes
- Cook time: 10 minutes

Ingredients

- 4 mahi-mahi fillets (4-6 oz each)
- 2 tbsp. olive oil
- 1/2 cup diced fresh pineapple
- 1/4 cup diced red onion
- 1 jalapeño pepper, seeded and diced
- 1 tbsp. fresh cilantro, chopped
- Salt and pepper to taste.

Nutrition information per serving

- Calories: 200
- Protein: 28g
- Fat: 9g
- Carbohydrates: 4g

Instructions

1. In a small bowl, mix together diced pineapple, red onion, jalapeño pepper, and cilantro.

2. Season mahi-mahi fillets with salt and pepper.

3. Over medium-high heat, heat a large skillet and add a small amount of oil.

4. Add mahi-mahi fillets to the skillet and cook for 3-4 minutes per side, or until the fish is cooked through and flakes easily with a fork.

5. Serve hot with a spoonful of pineapple salsa on top.

Health benefits: Mahi-mahi is a low-fat source of protein and a good source of vitamin B12, which is important for nerve and blood cell health.

Note_______________________________________

____

____

____

____

____

____

Your

Observation_______________________________________

____

____

____

____

____

Progress

Report_______________________________________

____

____

____

____

____

Poached Halibut in Coconut Curry Broth

Gently poach halibut fillets in a fragrant coconut curry broth infused with ginger, lemongrass, and turmeric for a flavorful low FODMAP dish.

- Serves: 4
- Prep time: 10 minutes
- Cook time: 20 minutes

Ingredients

- 4 halibut fillets (4-6 oz each)
- 1 can coconut milk
- 1 tbsp. red curry paste
- 1 tbsp. fresh ginger, grated
- 1 stalk lemongrass, chopped
- 1 tsp. ground turmeric
- Salt and pepper to taste.

Nutrition information per serving

- Calories: 290
- Protein: 34g
- Fat: 15g
- Carbohydrates: 4g

Instructions

1. In a large saucepan, whisk together coconut milk, red curry paste, ginger, lemongrass, and turmeric.

2. Season halibut fillets with salt and pepper, then add to the saucepan.

3. Bring the broth to a simmer and cook for 10-12 minutes, or until the fish is cooked through and flakes easily with a fork.

4. Serve hot with additional chopped cilantro, if desired.

Health benefits: Halibut is a lean source of protein and a good source of vitamin D, which is important for bone health.

Note____

____

____

____

____

____

Your

Observation________________________________

____

____

____

____

____

Progress

Report__________________________________

____

____

____

____

____

____

Herb-Crusted Baked Trout

Coat trout fillets in a mixture of gluten-free breadcrumbs and fresh herbs, then bake until the fish is golden and crispy on the outside.

- Serves: 4
- Prep time: 10 minutes
- Cook time: 15 minutes

Ingredients

- 4 trout fillets (4-6 oz each)
- 1/2 cup gluten-free breadcrumbs
- 1 tbsp. fresh parsley, chopped
- 1 tbsp. fresh thyme, chopped
- 1 tbsp. fresh rosemary, chopped
- 2 tbsp. olive oil
- Salt and pepper to taste

Nutrition information per serving

- Calories: 220
- Protein: 28g
- Fat: 9g
- Carbohydrates: 6g

Instructions
1. Preheat the oven to 400°F.

2. In a small bowl, mix together breadcrumbs, parsley, thyme, and rosemary.

3. Season trout fillets with salt and pepper, then brush with olive oil.

4. Coat the trout fillets with the breadcrumb mixture, pressing the mixture onto the fish to adhere.

5. Place trout fillets on a baking sheet and bake for 12-15 minutes, or until the fish is cooked through and the crust is golden and crispy.

6. Serve hot, if desired, with lemon wedges.

Health benefits: Trout is a good source of omega-3 fatty acids, which have been shown to reduce inflammation and improve heart health.

Note____

____

____

____

____

____

Your

Observation______________________________________

____

____

____

____

____

Progress

Report____

____

____

____

____

____

Egg Recipes

Soba Miso Soup with Jammy Eggs

Combine soba noodles, baby bok choy, oyster mushrooms, and perfectly cooked jammy eggs in a flavorful miso broth.

- Serves: 4
- Prep Time: 15 minutes
- Cook Time: 20 minutes

Ingredients

- 4 large eggs
- ½ cup dried soba noodles
- 1 bunch baby bok choy, chopped
- ¼ lb. shiitake mushrooms, sliced
- 4 cups vegetable stock
- 2 tbsp. white miso paste
- 1 tsp. grated fresh ginger
- 1 finely sliced green onion (only the green parts)
- 1 tbsp. sesame seeds
- Sea salt and black pepper, to taste

Nutritional Macros & Calories Per serving (without sesame seeds)

- Calories - 180 kcal

- Carbohydrate - 17g
- Protein - 12g
- Fat - 6g
- Fiber - 2g

Instructions

1. Place eggs in a medium pot filled with cold water; bring to a boil. Once boiling, remove from heat, cover, and set aside for 10 minutes. Run them under cool water until they reach room temperature. Peel and slice in half lengthwise.

2. Cook soba noodles according to package directions. Drain and rinse with cold water. Set aside.

3. Heat the vegetable stock in a separate pot over high heat. Add the ginger and simmer for 5 minutes. Reduce heat to low, then whisk in miso paste until dissolved.

4. In another pan, sauté mushrooms and bok choy with a pinch of salt until tender. Divide between four bowls.

5. Arrange soba noodles around the sides of the bowl. Pour hot miso soup over top.

6. Carefully place jammy egg halves atop the soup. Before serving, sprinkle with green onion and sesame seeds.

Health Benefits
- Rich in antioxidants and fiber from soba noodles and bok choy.
- Contains probiotics from miso paste, helping support healthy gut bacteria.
- Promotes satiety and nutrient absorption thanks to protein from eggs.

Note____

____

____

____

____

____

____

Your

Observation_____________________________________

____

____

____

____

____

Progress

Report____

____

____

____

____

____

Mini Frittatas

Create bite-sized frittatas customized with your favorite ingredients, ideal for freezing and enjoying throughout the week.

- Serves: 12 mini frittatas
- Prep Time: 15 minutes
- Cook Time: 20 minutes

Ingredients

- 12 large eggs
- ⅓ cup lactose-free milk or unsweetened almond milk
- ⅛ tsp garlic powder
- ⅛ tsp. onion powder
- ⅛ tsp. red pepper flakes
- ¾ cup diced bell peppers
- ¾ cup diced cherry tomatoes
- ½ cup finely chopped spinach
- ¼ cup minced shallots
- 2 tbsp. olive oil
- Sea salt and black pepper, to taste

Nutritional Macros & Calories Per mini frittata

- Calories - 65 kcal
- Carbohydrate - 2g
- Protein - 4g

- Fat - 5g
- Fiber - 0.5g

Instructions

1. Preheat the oven to 375°F (190°C). Coat a muffin tin with cooking spray.

2. Heat the olive oil in a skillet over medium heat. Add shallots and sauté until softened, approximately 3 minutes. Stir in bell peppers and cherry tomatoes, season lightly with salt and pepper, and continue cooking until veggies are slightly softened, about 5 more minutes. Remove from heat and let cool.

3. Whisk eggs, milk, garlic powder, onion powder, and red pepper flakes in a mixing bowl. Season with salt and pepper.

4. Evenly distribute the cooled vegetable mixture among the muffin cups. Top with spinach leaves.

5. Fill each cup almost full with the egg mixture.

6. Bake for 15–20 minutes, or until the edges are golden brown and the center is firm. Allow to cool slightly before removing from the muffin tray.

Health Benefits

- Packed with vitamin C and antioxidants from bell peppers and tomatoes.
- Offers a good source of iron and calcium from spinach.
- They are high in protein and low in crabs, making them a satisfying breakfast option.

Note____

____

____

____

____

____

Your

Observation_________________________________

____

____

____

____

____

Progress

Report______________________________________

____

____

____

____

____

Non-Alcoholic Egg Nog

Satisfy your festive cravings with delicious, non-alcoholic egg nog suitable for all ages.

- Serves: 4
- Prep Time: 10 minutes
- Cooking Time: 2 hours

Ingredients

- 4 large eggs, separated
- 2 cups unsweetened almond milk
- 1 tsp. vanilla extract
- 1 tsp. cinnamon
- ½ tsp ground nutmeg
- ¼ cup maple syrup
- ½ cup coconut cream
- Ice cubes

Nutritional Macros & Calories Per serving

- Calories - 220 kcal
- Carbohydrate - 15 g
- Protein - 8 g
- Fat - 16 g
- Fiber - 2 g

Instructions

1. Separate egg yolks and whites into two different mixing bowls.

2. Beat egg yolks with almond milk, vanilla extract, cinnamon, nutmeg, and maple syrup until smooth.

3. Using clean beaters, whip egg whites until stiff peaks form.

4. Gradually fold the beaten egg whites into the egg yolk mixture.

5. Chill the mixture in the refrigerator for at least two hours.

6. To serve, pour equal amounts of eggnog into glasses filled with ice cubes. Grate fresh nutmeg overtop if desired.

Health Benefits

- Loaded with essential amino acids from eggs.
- Boosts immunity with antioxidants from spices like cinnamon and nutmeg.
- Lower in sugar compared to traditional eggnog made with cows milk and added sugars.

Note____

____

____

____

____

____

____

Your

Observation___________________________________

____

____

____

____

____

____

Progress

Report___________________________________

____

____

____

____

____

Bacon Deviled Eggs

Transform ordinary hard-boiled eggs into a delectable appetizer featuring smoked bacon.

- Serves: 6
- Prep Time: 15 minutes
- Cook Time: 15 minutes

Ingredients

- 6 large eggs
- 2 strips uncured nitrate-free bacon
- 2 tbsp. mayonnaise
- 1 tsp Dijon mustard
- 1 tsp. apple cider vinegar
- ⅛ tsp. paprika
- Sea salt and black pepper, to taste
- Fresh chives, chopped, for garnish

Nutritional Macros & Calories Per serving (2 deviled egg halves)

- Calories - 120 kcal
- Carbohydrate - 1g
- Protein - 7g
- Fat - 10g
- Fiber - 0g

Instructions

1. Place eggs in a medium pot filled with cold water; bring to a boil. Once boiling, remove from heat, cover, and set aside for 10 minutes. Run them under cool water until they reach room temperature. Peel and slice in half lengthwise.

2. Cook the bacon in a pan over medium heat until crisp. Remove from the pan and chop into small pieces.

3. Remove the yolks from the egg halves and place them in a mixing bowl. Add mayonnaise, Dijon mustard, apple cider vinegar, paprika, salt, and pepper. Mash it with a fork until smooth.

4. Spoon or pipe the yolk mixture back into the egg white halves.

5. Top each deviled egg with chopped bacon and fresh chives.

Health Benefits

- Provides a good source of protein and healthy fats from eggs and bacon.
- They are low in crabs and high in flavor, making them a satisfying snack or appetizer.
- Contains choline, a nutrient important for brain health, found in egg yolks.

Note____

____

____

____

____

____

Your

Observation_______________________________________

____

____

____

____

____

Progress

Report_______________________________________

____

____

____

____

____

Italian Meringue Buttercream

Craft a sophisticated frosting for your desserts, utilizing egg whites for a lighter texture.

- Serves: 12
- Prep Time: 15 minutes
- Cook Time: 10 minutes

Ingredients

- 4 large egg whites
- 1 cup granulated sugar
- ¼ cup water
- 1 cup unsalted butter, softened
- 1 tsp. vanilla extract

Nutritional Macros & Calories Per serving (2 tbsp)

Calories - 140 kcal
- Carbohydrate - 12g
- Protein - 0g
- Fat - 10g
- Fiber - 0g

Instructions

1. In a mixing bowl, beat egg whites until stiff peaks form.

2. In a saucepan, combine sugar and water. Heat over medium-high heat until the mixture reaches 240°F (115°C) on a candy thermometer.

3. With the mixer running on low speed, slowly pour the hot sugar syrup into the egg whites.

4. Increase the mixer speed to high and continue beating until the mixture cools to room temperature.

5. Add softened butter and vanilla extract to the mixing bowl. Beat until smooth and creamy.

Health Benefits

- Contains healthy fats from butter, which can help improve cholesterol levels.
- Low in sugar compared to traditional buttercream recipes.
- Provides a source of protein from egg whites.

Note____

____

____

____

____

____

____

Your

Observation_______________________________________

____

____

____

____

____

Progress

Report____

____

____

____

____

____

Butterscotch Pudding with Salted Caramel Sauce

Indulge in a comforting treat with a hint of sea salt, complementing the rich butterscotch flavor.

- Serves: 4
- Prep Time: 10 minutes
- Cook Time: 20 minutes

Ingredients

- 4 large egg yolks
- 2 cups lactose-free or unsweetened almond milk
- ½ cup brown sugar
- 2 tbsp. cornstarch
- 1 tsp. vanilla extract
- ¼ tsp sea salt
- 2 tbsp. unsalted butter
- 2 tbsp. maple syrup
- ¼ tsp sea salt

Nutritional Macros & Calories Per serving

- Calories - 250 kcal
- Carbohydrate - 35 g
- Protein - 6 g
- Fat - 10 g

- Fiber - 0 g

Instructions

1. In a mixing bowl, whisk together egg yolks, milk, brown sugar, cornstarch, vanilla extract, and sea salt.

2. Pour the mixture into a saucepan and cook over medium heat, stirring constantly, until it thickens and coats the back of a spoon, about 10 minutes.

3. Remove from heat and stir in butter until melted and smooth.

4. Divide the pudding among four serving dishes and chill in the refrigerator for at least 1 hour.

5. In a separate saucepan, heat maple syrup and sea salt over medium heat until it begins to bubble and thicken, about 5 minutes.

6. Drizzle salted caramel sauce over chilled pudding before serving.

Health Benefits

- Milk provides a good source of calcium and vitamin D.
- Contains healthy fats from egg yolks and butter.

- Lower in sugar compared to traditional butterscotch pudding recipes.

"SIBO-friendly cooking made simple—enjoy flavorful meals without the worry."

Note____

____

____

____

____

____

Your

Observation______________________________________

____

____

____

____

____

Progress

Report____

____

____

____

____

____

Go-To Low FODMAP Breakfast

Start your day right with a hearty egg scramble packed with roasted potatoes, leafy greens, and turkey sausage crumbles.

- Serves: 2
- Prep Time: 10 minutes
- Cook Time: 15 minutes

Ingredients

- 4 large eggs
- 2 tbsp. lactose-free milk or unsweetened almond milk
- 1 tbsp. olive oil
- 1 cup diced roasted potatoes
- 1 cup baby spinach leaves
- 2 turkey sausage links, crumbled
- Sea salt and black pepper, to taste

Nutritional Macros & Calories Per serving

- Calories - 280 kcal
- Carbohydrate - 14 g
- Protein - 18 g
- Fat - 16 g
- Fiber - 2 g

Instructions

1. Whisk the eggs and milk in a mixing bowl. Season with salt and pepper.

2. Heat olive oil over medium heat in a skillet. Add diced potatoes and cook until crispy, about 5 minutes.

3. Add baby spinach leaves and turkey sausage crumbles to the skillet. Cook for approximately 3 minutes, or until the spinach has wilted.

4. Pour the egg mixture over the potato mixture. Cook, stirring occasionally, until eggs are set, about 5 minutes.

Health Benefits

- It is high in protein and low in crabs, making it a satisfying breakfast option.
- It provides a good source of iron and vitamin C from spinach.
- Contains healthy fats from olive oil.

Note_______________________________________

____

____

____

____

____

Your

Observation_______________________________

____

____

____

____

____

Progress

Report_______________________________________

____

____

____

____

____

Ultimate Low FODMAP Frittata

Wake up to a colorful frittata bursting with roasted vegetables, feta, and spinach.

- Serves: 6
- Prep Time: 15 minutes
- Cook Time: 25 minutes

Ingredients

- 8 large eggs
- 2 tbsp. lactose-free milk or unsweetened almond milk
- 1 tbsp. olive oil
- 1 cup diced roasted sweet potatoes
- 1 cup diced red bell peppers
- 1 cup baby spinach leaves
- ½ cup crumbled feta cheese
- Sea salt and black pepper, to taste

Nutritional Macros & Calories Per serving

- Calories - 180 kcal
- Carbohydrate - 8g
- Protein - 11g
- Fat - 11g
- Fiber - 2g

Instructions

1. Preheat the oven to 375°F (190°C).

2. Whisk the eggs and milk in a mixing bowl. Season with salt and pepper.

3. Heat olive oil in a skillet over medium heat. Add diced sweet potatoes and cook until slightly softened, about 5 minutes.

4. Add diced red bell peppers and baby spinach leaves to the skillet. Cook until the spinach is wilted, about 3 minutes.

5. Pour the egg mixture over the vegetable mixture. Sprinkle feta cheese over top.

6. Bake in the oven for 20–25 minutes, or until the center is set and the edges are golden brown.

Health Benefits

- Provides a good source of vitamin A and potassium from sweet potatoes.
- Contains antioxidants and vitamin C from red bell peppers.
- It is high in protein and low in carbs, making it a satisfying meal option.

Note___________________________________

____

____

____

____

____

Your

Observation___________________________________

____

____

____

____

____

____

Progress

Report___________________________________

____

____

____

____

____

Egg Shakshuka

Experience Middle Eastern cuisine with a twist, combining poached eggs with a zesty tomato sauce.

- Serves: 4
- Prep Time: 10 minutes
- Cook Time: 25 minutes

Ingredients

- 4 large eggs
- 1 can (14 oz) diced tomatoes
- 1 red bell pepper, diced
- 1 small zucchini, diced
- 1/2 cup chopped fresh parsley
- 2 tbsp. olive oil
- 2 tsp. ground cumin
- 1 tsp. smoked paprika
- 1/2 tsp. cayenne pepper
- Salt and black pepper, to taste

Nutritional Macros & Calories Per serving

- Calories - 180 kcal
- Carbohydrate - 10 g
- Protein - 10 g
- Fat - 12 g
- Fiber - 3 g

Instructions

1. Heat olive oil in a large skillet over medium heat. Add diced bell pepper and zucchini. Sauté until softened, about 5 minutes.

2. Stir in ground cumin, smoked paprika, and cayenne pepper. Cook for an additional minute.

3. Pour in the diced tomatoes and season with salt and black pepper. Simmer for 10 minutes.

4. Using a spoon, create small wells in the tomato mixture. Crack an egg into each well.

5. Cover the skillet and cook until the egg whites are set but the yolks are still runny, about 5-7 minutes.

6. Sprinkle with chopped parsley before serving.

Health Benefits

- Tomatoes are rich in lycopene and vitamin C.
- Provides a good source of vitamin A and antioxidants from bell peppers.
- It is high in protein and low in crabs, making it a satisfying meal option.

Note____

____

____

____

____

____

____

Your

Observation_______________________________________

____

____

____

____

____

Progress

Report____

____

____

____

____

____

Low FODMAP Baked Egg Cups

Prepare a versatile dish that can be adapted to suit various tastes, offering convenience and variety.

- Serves: 6
- Prep Time: 10 minutes
- Cook Time: 20 minutes

Ingredients

- 6 large eggs
- 1/2 cup diced red bell pepper
- 1/2 cup diced zucchini
- 1/4 cup chopped chives
- 1/4 cup chopped spinach
- Salt and black pepper, to taste

Nutritional Macros & Calories Per serving (1 egg cup)

- Calories - 70 kcal
- Carbohydrate - 2g
- Protein - 6g
- Fat - 4g
- Fiber - 0.5g

Instructions

1. Preheat the oven to 350°F (175°C). With cooking spray, grease a muffin tin.

2. In a large bowl, whisk the eggs. Stir in the red bell pepper, zucchini, chives, and spinach. Season with salt and black pepper.

3. Pour the egg mixture into the prepared muffin cups, filling them about three-quarters full.

4. Bake in the preheated oven until the egg cups are set, about 15-20 minutes.

Health Benefits

- Packed with vitamin C and antioxidants from red bell peppers.
- Offers a good source of vitamin K and iron from spinach.
- They are high in protein and low in crabs, making them a satisfying breakfast option.

Note

Your

Observation

Progress

Report

Meat Recipes

Grilled Chicken Skewers

Marinate chicken in a mixture of olive oil, lemon juice, garlic-infused oil, and herbs. Thread on skewers and heat until cooked through.

- Serves: 4
- Prep Time: 15 minutes
- Cook Time: 10–15 minutes

Ingredients

- 1 pound boneless, skinless chicken breast, cut into bite-sized pieces.
- ¼ cup olive oil
- 2 tbsp. freshly squeezed lemon juice
- 1 tsp. garlic-infused oil
- Salt and pepper to taste
- Wooden skewers (soaked in water if wooden)

Nutritional Macros per serving (approximate)

- Calories: 210 kcal
- Protein: 32g
- Fat: 9g
- Carbohydrate: 1g

- Sugar: 0g
- Fiber: 0g

Instructions

1. Prepare the marinade by combining olive oil, lemon juice, garlic-infused oil, salt, and pepper in a bowl.

2. Add the chicken pieces to the marinade and mix thoroughly. Cover and chill for at least 30 minutes.

3. Preheat the grill to medium heat.

4. Thread the chicken evenly onto skewers.

5. Place skewers on a preheated grill and cook for approximately 5 minutes on each side, or until internal temperature reaches 165°F (74°C).

Health Benefits: Chicken is rich in protein, vitamins, and minerals essential for maintaining muscle mass, bone strength, and immune function. Olive oil contains healthy monounsaturated fats and antioxidants, while lemons offer vitamin C and fiber.

Note____

____

____

____

____

Your

Observation______________________________________

____

____

____

____

Progress

Report______________________________________

____

____

____

____

____

Beef Stir-Fry

Sauté beef strips with low FODMAP vegetables such as bok choy, carrots, and bell peppers. Season with sesame oil, ginger, and soy sauce.

- Serves: 4
- Prep Time: 15 minutes
- Cook Time: 10 minutes

Ingredients

- 1 lb. lean beef sirloin steak, thinly sliced
- ½ head broccoli, chopped into bite-size florets
- 1 large carrot, julienned
- 1 red bell pepper, sliced
- 2 cloves garlic, minced (or use garlic-infused oil)
- 2 tbsp. reduced sodium soy sauce
- 1 tbsp. sesame oil
- Salt and pepper to taste

Nutritional Macros per serving (approximate)

- Calories: 220 kcal
- Protein: 25g
- Fat: 10g
- Carbohydrate: 10g
- Sugar: 5g
- Fiber: 3g

Instructions

1. Heat a nonstick skillet or wok over high heat.

2. Add the beef and stir-fry until lightly browned, about 2 minutes. Remove the beef from the pan and set it aside.

3. In the same pan, add sesame oil and sauté garlic until fragrant, about 30 seconds.

4. Add broccoli, carrots, and bell peppers; season with salt and pepper. Stir-fry until crisp-tender, about 2 minutes.

5. Return the steak to the pan, along with the soy sauce. Continue cooking until heated through, about 1 minute more.

Health Benefits: Lean beef provides iron, zinc, and B vitamins important for energy production and cellular repair. Cruciferous veggies like broccoli contain sulforaphane, a compound shown to support detoxification pathways and promote heart health.

Note____

____

____

____

____

____

____

Your

Observation_______________________________________

____

____

____

____

____

____

Progress

Report_______________________________________

____

____

____

____

____

____

Turkey Meatballs

Mix ground turkey with gluten-free breadcrumbs, eggs, and herbs. Bake in the oven and serve with low FODMAP tomato sauce.

- Serves: 4
- Prep Time: 15 minutes
- Cook Time: 20 minutes

Ingredients

- 1 lb. extra-lean ground turkey
- ⅓ cup gluten-free breadcrumbs
- 1 large egg
- 1 tbsp. dried parsley
- 1 tsp. dried basil
- ½ tsp salt
- ⅛ tsp. black pepper

Nutritional Macros per serving (approximate)

- Calories: 180 kcal
- Protein: 25 g
- Fat: 6 g
- Carbohydrate: 6 g
- Sugar: 1 g
- Fiber: 1 g

Instructions

1. Preheat the oven to 375°F (190°C). Line the baking sheet with parchment paper.

2. Combine all ingredients in a mixing bowl. Use your hands to gently combine without overworking the mixture.

3. Form the mixture into golf ball-sized balls and place them on the lined baking sheet.

4. Bake for 15–20 minutes or until internal temperature reaches 165°F (74°C).

Health Benefits: Ground turkey offers similar nutrients to beef but with fewer calories and less saturated fat. Gluten-free breadcrumbs help bind the meatballs without adding unnecessary crabs.

Note____

____

____

____

____

____

____

Your

Observation_______________________________________

____

____

____

____

____

____

Progress

Report_______________________________________

____

____

____

____

____

____

Pork Tenderloin

Rub pork tenderloin with a mixture of paprika, cumin, and oregano. Roast in the oven until fully done.

- Serves: 4
- Prep Time: 10 minutes
- Cook Time: 20 minutes

Ingredients

- 1 lb. pork tenderloin
- 1 tsp. paprika
- 1 tsp. cumin
- 1 tsp. dried oregano
- Salt and pepper to taste

Nutritional Macros per serving (approximate)

- Calories: 160 kcal
- Protein: 28g
- Fat: 4g
- Carbohydrate: 1g
- Sugar: 0g
- Fiber: 0g

Instructions

1. Preheat the oven to 375°F (190°C).

2. Pat dry pork tenderloin and rub spices evenly over the surface.

3. Place pork tenderloin on a roasting rack placed inside a shallow baking dish.

4. Roast for 20 minutes, or until internal temperature reaches 145°F (63°C), allowing for a 5-minute resting period before cutting.

Health Benefits: Pork tenderloin is a good source of protein and B vitamins, including niacin and thiamin, which play crucial roles in energy production and nervous system function. The spices used in this recipe may aid in reducing inflammation and improving blood circulation.

Note_______________________________

____

____

____

____

____

Your

Observation_______________________

____

____

____

____

____

Progress

Report__________________________

____

____

____

____

____

Lamb Chops

Season lamb chops with rosemary, thyme, and garlic-infused oil. Grill until cooked to your liking.

- Serves: 4
- Prep Time: 5 minutes
- Cook Time: 10 minutes

Ingredients

- 8 lamb loin chops
- 1 tsp. dried rosemary
- 1 tsp. dried thyme
- 2 tbsp. garlic-infused oil*
- Salt and pepper to taste

Nutritional Macros per serving (approximate)

- Calories: 280 kcal
- Protein: 25g
- Fat: 18g
- Carbohydrate: 0g
- Sugar: 0g
- Fiber: 0g

Instructions

1. Preheat the grill to medium-high heat.

2. In a small bowl, combine rosemary, thyme, garlic-infused oil, salt, and pepper.

3. Rub the mixture on both sides of the lamb chops.

4. Grill the chops for about 5 minutes on each side for medium-rare, or to your desired level of doneness.

Health Benefits: Lamb is an excellent source of high-quality protein and essential nutrients such as iron and zinc. The herbs and garlic-infused oil not only enhance the flavor but also offer potential anti-inflammatory and antimicrobial properties.

Note

Your

Observation

Progress

Report

Beef and Broccoli

Sauté beef strips with broccoli and green beans. Season with sesame oil, ginger, and soy sauce.

- Serves: 4
- Prep Time: 15 minutes
- Cook Time: 10 minutes

Ingredients

- 1 lb. beef sirloin, thinly sliced
- 1 head broccoli, cut into florets
- 1 cup green beans, trimmed
- 2 tbsp. reduced sodium soy sauce
- 1 tsp. fresh ginger, grated
- 1 tbsp. sesame oil
- Salt and pepper to taste

Nutritional Macros per serving (approximate)

- Calories: 250 kcal
- Protein: 30g
- Fat: 10g
- Carbohydrate: 10g
- Sugar: 3g
- Fiber: 4g

Instructions

1. In a bowl, combine soy sauce, ginger, and sesame oil. Add the beef slices, and let them marinate for at least 10 minutes.

2. Heat a big skillet or wok over high heat. Add beef and stir-fry until browned. Remove from the pan and set aside.

3. Add a little extra oil to the same pan if needed. Stir-fry broccoli and green beans until tender-crisp.

4. Return the beef to the pan, add the soy sauce mixture, and toss to combine. Cook for an additional minute.

Health Benefits: This dish provides a good balance of protein, fiber, and essential nutrients. Broccoli and green beans are rich in vitamins C and K, as well as folate and fiber, while beef offers high-quality protein and important minerals like iron and zinc.

Note

Your

Observation

Progress

Report

Chicken Curry

Cook chicken in a low FODMAP curry sauce made with coconut milk, turmeric, and cumin. Serve over rice or gluten-free naan bread.

- Serves: 4
- Prep Time: 15 minutes
- Cook Time: 25 minutes

Ingredients

- 1 pound of boneless, skinless chicken breast, sliced into bite-sized pieces
- 1 can (14 oz) coconut milk
- 2 tbsp. low FODMAP curry powder
- 1 tsp. ground turmeric
- 1 tsp. ground cumin
- Salt to taste

Nutritional Macros per serving (approximate)

- Calories: 320 kcal
- Protein: 30g
- Fat: 20 g
- Carbohydrate: 6g
- Sugar: 2g
- Fiber: 2g

Instructions

1. In a large skillet, heat a small amount of oil over medium heat. Add chicken pieces and cook until no longer pink.

2. Stir in curry powder, turmeric, and cumin; cook for an additional minute.

3. Pour in the coconut milk and bring to a gentle simmer. Cook for around 15-20 minutes, or until the chicken is fully cooked and the sauce has thickened.

Health Benefits: Chicken is an excellent source of lean protein, while coconut milk provides healthy fats and a creamy texture without lactose. The spices used in this recipe offer potential anti-inflammatory properties and may aid indigestion.

Note____

____

____

____

____

____

Your

Observation_______________________________________

____

____

____

____

____

Progress

Report____

____

____

____

____

____

Turkey Burgers

Mix ground turkey with grated zucchini, eggs, and herbs. Grill and serve on a gluten-free bun with low FODMAP toppings such as lettuce and tomato.

- Serves: 4
- Prep Time: 15 minutes
- Cook Time: 10 minutes

Ingredients

- 1 lb. ground turkey
- 1 medium zucchini, grated
- 1 large egg
- 2 tbsp. chopped fresh parsley
- 1 tsp. dried oregano
- Salt and pepper to taste
- Gluten-free buns
- Low FODMAP toppings (lettuce, tomato, etc.)

Nutritional Macros per serving (approximate)

- Calories: 220 kcal
- Protein: 25g
- Fat: 10g
- Carbohydrate: 10g
- Sugar: 2g
- Fiber: 2g

Instructions

1. In a large bowl, combine ground turkey, grated zucchini, egg, parsley, oregano, salt, and pepper.

2. Mix well and form into 4 patties.

3. Heat a grill or grill pan over medium-high heat. Cook the burgers for about 5 minutes per side, or until fully done.

4. Serve on gluten-free buns with low FODMAP toppings of your choice.

Health Benefits: Ground turkey is a lean protein source that is lower in saturated fat than beef. Zucchini adds fiber and vitamins, while fresh herbs provide flavor and potential health benefits.

Note

Your

Observation

Progress

Report

Pork Ribs

Rub the pork ribs with a mixture of smoked paprika, cumin, and brown sugar. Slowly cook in the oven until tender.

- Serves: 4
- Prep Time: 10 minutes
- Cook Time: 2 hours

Ingredients

- 2 lbs. pork ribs
- 1 tbsp. smoked paprika
- 1 tsp. ground cumin
- 1 tbsp. brown sugar
- Salt and pepper to taste

Nutritional Macros per serving (approximate)

- Calories: 400 kcal
- Protein: 30g
- Fat: 30g
- Carbohydrate: 5g
- Sugar: 4g
- Fiber: 0g

Instructions

1. Preheat the oven to 300°F (150°C).

2. In a small bowl, mix together smoked paprika, cumin, brown sugar, salt, and pepper.

3. Rub the spice mixture all over the pork ribs.

4. Place the ribs on a baking sheet and bake for 2 hours, or until tender.

Health Benefits: Pork ribs are a good source of protein and essential nutrients like iron and zinc. Smoked paprika adds flavor and potential antioxidant benefits.

"Goodbye discomfort, hello deliciousness— transforms your meals with this cookbook."

Note

Your

Observation

Progress

Report

Lamb Kebabs

Marinate lamb cubes in a mixture of olive oil, lemon juice, and herbs. Thread onto skewers with low FODMAP vegetables such as zucchini and bell peppers. Grill until cooked through.

- Serves: 4
- Prep Time: 15 minutes
- Cook Time: 10 minutes

Ingredients

- 1 lb. lamb leg meat, cut into cubes
- 1 medium zucchini, sliced
- 1 red bell pepper, cut into chunks
- 1 tbsp. olive oil
- 1 tbsp. freshly squeezed lemon juice
- 1 tsp. dried oregano
- Salt and pepper to taste

Nutritional Macros per serving (approximate)

- Calories: 280 kcal
- Protein: 25g
- Fat: 16g
- Carbohydrate: 6g
- Sugar: 3g
- Fiber: 2g

Instructions

1. Preheat the grill to medium-high heat.

2. In a small bowl, whisk together olive oil, lemon juice, oregano, salt, and pepper.

3. Thread lamb, zucchini, and bell pepper onto skewers.

4. Brush the skewers with olive oil mixture.

5. Grill the skewers for about 5 minutes on each side, or until the lamb is cooked to your liking.

Health Benefits: Lamb is a good source of protein and essential nutrients like iron and vitamin B12. Zucchini and bell pepper add fiber and vitamins, while olive oil provides healthy fats and antioxidants.

"Flavorful solutions, gut-friendly delights."

Note____

____

____

____

____

____

Your

Observation_______________________________________

____

____

____

____

____

Progress

Report_______________________________________

____

____

____

____

____

Meal plan

BLD	*DAY 1*	*DAY 2*	*DAY 3*
Breakfast	GoTo Low FODMAP Breakfast	Mini Frittatas	Low FODMAP Baked Egg Cups
Lunch	Tuna Salad Lettuce Wraps	Egg Shakshuka	Turkey Burgers
Dinner	Grilled Salmon with Lemon and Dill	Baked Cod with Herbs	PanSeared Tilapia with Cilantro Lime Butter

BLD	*DAY 4*	*DAY 5*	*DAY 6*
Breakfast	Soba Miso Soup with Jammy Eggs	Ultimate Low FODMAP Frittata	Non-Alcoholic Egg Nog
Lunch	Chicken Curry	Beef Stir-fry	Turkey Meatballs
Dinner	Dinner: Lemon Garlic Shrimp Skewers	Grilled Swordfish Steaks with Herb Marinade	Baked Haddock with Tomato and Olive Salsa

BLD	DAY 7	DAY 8	DAY 9
Breakfast	Egg Shakshuka	Mini Frittatas	GoTo Low FODMAP Breakfast
Lunch	Pork Ribs	Lamb Kebabs	Beef and Broccoli
Dinner	Seared Mahi Mahi with Pineapple Salsa	Poached Halibut in Coconut Curry Broth	Herb Crusted Baked Trout

BLD	DAY 10	DAY 11	DAY 12
Breakfast	Low FODMAP Baked Egg Cups	Mini Frittatas	Soba Miso Soup with Jammy Eggs
Lunch	Chicken Curry	Turkey Burgers	Beef Stir-fry
Dinner	Grilled Salmon with Lemon and Dill	Baked Cod with Herbs	Lemon Garlic Shrimp Skewers

BLD	DAY 13	DAY 14	DAY 15
Breakfast	Non-Alcoholic Egg Nog	Ultimate Low FODMAP Frittata	Egg Shakshuka
Lunch	Pork Tenderloin	Lamb Chops	Turkey Meatballs
Dinner	Pan Seared Tilapia with Cilantro Lime Butter	Grilled Swordfish Steaks with Herb Marinade	Baked Haddock with Tomato and Olive Salsa

BLD	DAY 16	DAY 17	DAY 18
Breakfast	GoTo Low FODMAP Breakfast	Low FODMAP Baked Egg Cups	Mini Frittatas
Lunch	Chicken Curry	Beef and Broccoli	Pork Ribs
Dinner	Seared Mahi Mahi with Pineapple Salsa	Herb Crusted Baked Trout	Poached Halibut in Coconut Curry Broth

BLD	DAY 19	DAY 20	DAY 21
Breakfast	Soba Miso Soup with Jammy Eggs	Non-Alcoholic Egg Nog	Ultimate Low FODMAP Frittata
Lunch	Lamb Kebabs	Beef Stir-fry	Turkey Burgers
Dinner	Grilled Salmon with Lemon and Dill	Lemon Garlic Shrimp Skewers	Baked Cod with Herbs

Hope the book is Useful if Yes; Please Kindly Leave Your Honest Review Thank!!!!!

www.ingramcontent.com/pod-product-compliance
Lightning Source LLC
Chambersburg PA
CBHW070817280726
48660CB00016B/2045